Modern Guide To Say No To IBS

A Comprehensive Guide To Understanding, Managing, And Supporting Individuals With Irritable Bowel Syndrome (IBS)

Nora B. Payne

Table Of Contents

Introduction

Irritable Bowel Syndrome profoundly affects persons emotionally, producing stress, worry, and diminished quality of life. The unexpected nature of symptoms, social barriers, and the chronicity of the illness add to mental anguish. Addressing the emotional toll is key for comprehensive IBS care and promoting overall well-being.

Chronic gastrointestinal illness, often known as irritable bowel syndrome (IBS), is a condition that affects millions of individuals all over the world. It causes disruptions in their everyday lives and has an impact on their general well-being. Abdominal discomfort, bloating, and irregular bowel movements are some of the symptoms that are associated with this disorder of the digestive tract. Irritable bowel syndrome (IBS) manifests itself due to several circumstances, although the specific etiology of the condition is still unknown. Because the diagnosis of irritable bowel syndrome (IBS) is dependent on the presence of distinctive symptoms and the exclusion of other digestive illnesses, it is sometimes difficult to perform. When diagnosing irritable bowel syndrome (IBS), the Rome criteria, which is a collection of recommendations created by medical professionals, is frequently utilized.

Individuals who suffer from irritable bowel syndrome (IBS) frequently feel physical discomfort, psychological and emotional anguish, as well as increased stress and worry. Therefore, it is essential to provide appropriate treatment and management to meet the numerous problems that are offered by IBS. It is very necessary to take a comprehensive approach to care, which includes not only medical interventions but also alterations to lifestyle and mental support. Effective management of IBS needs a joint effort between healthcare providers, patients with IBS, and their support networks. By recognizing the necessity of adequate treatment, we may pave the way for greater symptom management, enhanced quality of life, and a more profound feeling of well-being for people navigating the difficulties of IBS.

In the following parts, we will investigate the subtleties of IBS, and evaluate its symptoms, causes, demographic variables, and potential ramifications when left mismanaged. Practical solutions for managing and decreasing the burden of IBS will be explored, stressing the relevance of a healthy lifestyle in lowering the likelihood of getting the illness.

This is a thorough reference that attempts to give information, tactics, and insights for successful management and better well-being. The book focuses on education and awareness for persons diagnosed with IBS, as well as caregivers and support networks. It gives practical ways for controlling symptoms, including medication therapies, lifestyle adjustments, and stress management approaches.

The book also highlights the significance of a healthy lifestyle in avoiding and controlling IBS, highlighting particular habits like not smoking, regular exercise, proper sleep, and a balanced diet. By incorporating these factors into daily life, individuals might potentially minimize their risk and boost general well-being.

The book demystifies the complexities of IBS by offering accurate information, eliminating myths, and fostering a nuanced knowledge of the illness. It argues for a holistic approach to IBS care, understanding the interdependence of physical and emotional well-being. Addressing the physiological and psychological components of IBS can lead to a more balanced and meaningful existence.

The book underlines the necessity of emotional support, both from healthcare experts and personal networks, in managing the emotional issues associated with IBS. In short, "Navigating Wellness" aspires to be a beacon of support, understanding, and direction for people impacted by IBS and those devoted to giving care and assistance. Through educated information and caring insights, it strives to contribute to a path of greater well-being and resilience for persons living with Irritable Bowel Syndrome.

Understanding Irritable Bowel Syndrome (IBS)

Irritable Bowel Syndrome (IBS) is a complicated gastrointestinal condition that substantially disrupts the lives of individuals affected. This section seeks to give a full overview of IBS, diving into its description, many kinds, and the intricate interplay of variables leading to its emergence.

Definition and Explanation of IBS

Irritable Bowel Syndrome is a functional gastrointestinal condition defined by a constellation of symptoms affecting the digestive tract. Unlike other gastrointestinal diseases, IBS does not cause structural damage to the digestive organs but disturbs their regular functioning. The characteristic symptoms of IBS include stomach pain or discomfort, abnormal bowel habits (diarrhea, constipation, or a combination of both), and bloating. The diagnosis of IBS is typically complicated, based on the presence of distinctive symptoms and the exclusion of other gastrointestinal illnesses.

Understanding IBS entails knowing that it is a chronic disorder, meaning patients may endure symptoms throughout their life. The shifting pattern of symptoms can be unexpected, impacting daily activities and overall quality of life.

Types of IBS (e.g., IBS-D, IBS-C, IBS-M)

IBS presents in many kinds, each defined by specific patterns of bowel movements. These subtypes include:

1. IBS-D (Diarrhea-major): Individuals with IBS-D report frequent episodes of diarrhea as a major symptom.

2. IBS-C (Constipation-Predominant): This subtype involves infrequent and difficult bowel motions, with constipation being the main symptom.

3. IBS-M (Mixed): IBS-M contains symptoms of both IBS-D and IBS-C, resulting in a fluctuation between diarrhea and constipation.

Understanding these categories is critical for designing management techniques to target individual symptoms and enhance overall symptom control.

Causes and Triggers

Unraveling the subtleties of what causes IBS entails evaluating a mix of variables, both physiological and environmental. While the actual origin remains mysterious, numerous factors contribute to the appearance of IBS symptoms.

1. Role of Oversensitive Nerves

Oversensitive nerves in the gastrointestinal system play a crucial role in the development of IBS symptoms. The gut-brain axis, a complex communication network between the stomach and the brain, is considered to be dysregulated in persons with IBS. This imbalance can lead to heightened sensitivity to typical digestive processes, resulting in pain and discomfort.

2. Influence of Stress

Stress is a well-documented cause of IBS symptoms. The intimate relationship between the brain and the stomach implies that emotional and psychological pressures can increase symptoms. Chronic stress can lead to the worsening of stomach discomfort, bloating, and abnormalities in bowel patterns.

3. Genetic Factors

Genetics also have a role in predisposing persons to IBS. Studies have revealed that a family history of IBS might increase the probability of having the disorder. While precise genetic markers are currently under research, the hereditary component sheds light on the intricacy of IBS pathogenesis.

4. Other Environmental Factors

Beyond genetics, several environmental variables might contribute to the onset or worsening of IBS. These include

Dietary Habits: Certain meals, such as those heavy in fat, spice, or artificial sweeteners, may provoke symptoms in vulnerable individuals.

Gut Microbiota: Imbalances in the gut microbiota, the varied population of bacteria dwelling in the digestive system, have been associated with IBS. Disruptions in this delicate equilibrium may contribute to symptom onset.

Infections: Gastrointestinal infections can serve as a triggering cause for IBS, with symptoms lingering after the infection has gone.

Understanding the varied nature of these causes and triggers is vital for creating comprehensive and tailored methods for managing and minimizing the impact of

IBS. In the future sections, we will investigate the demographic variables determining IBS, the possible repercussions of uncontrolled IBS, and solutions for successful care and lifestyle adjustments.

Symptoms of Irritable Bowel Syndrome

Irritable Bowel Syndrome (IBS) emerges via a range of symptoms, creating a daunting terrain for both persons suffering from the disorder and healthcare providers attempting to offer effective therapy. This section tries to give a comprehensive study of the common symptoms associated with IBS, highlighting the diversity and severity that define this illness.

Common Symptoms

Understanding the symptoms of IBS is critical for quick diagnosis and appropriate care. IBS symptoms can vary greatly among individuals, and the prevalence of one or more of these symptoms over an extended time generally motivates individuals to seek medical assistance.

1. Abdominal Pain

Abdominal discomfort is a defining symptom of IBS, typically characterized as crampy or severe. The discomfort is often present in the lower abdomen and may be eased or aggravated by bowel motions. The severity and duration of stomach discomfort might change, contributing to the unpredictable character of IBS.

For many patients with IBS, stomach discomfort profoundly disrupts daily functioning and quality of life. The discomfort may range from moderate to severe, and its persistence can lead to heightened worry and stress, further increasing symptoms.

2. Bloating

Bloating is a frequent symptom in patients with IBS and is characterized by a sense of abdominal fullness or distention. This feeling is not necessarily connected to increased gas production but rather to altered gut motility and sensitivity. Bloating can lead to physical pain and influence body image and self-esteem.

Understanding the reasons for bloating, such as specific food choices or stress, is vital for persons looking to manage this condition efficiently. Addressing dietary issues, practicing relaxation techniques, and understanding personal triggers might lead to improved bloating management.

3. Diarrhea

Diarrhea is a frequent sign of IBS, particularly in persons with the diarrhea-predominant subtype (IBS-D). Frequent loose or watery stools, urgency to have a bowel movement, and an irregular bowel pattern define this symptom. The impact of diarrhea extends beyond the bodily component, impacting social and emotional well-being.

Managing diarrhea in IBS needs a complex strategy, including dietary alterations, medication management, and lifestyle improvements. Identifying particular factors that aggravate diarrhea helps individuals to proactively limit the burden on everyday life.

4. Constipation

In contrast to diarrhea, constipation is a prominent symptom in the constipation-predominant subtype of IBS (IBS-C). Individuals with IBS-C may suffer infrequent bowel movements, straining during bowel movements, and a sensation of incomplete evacuation. Constipation can lead to abdominal pain and influence overall gastrointestinal function.

Effective therapy of constipation requires dietary modifications, proper hydration consumption, and, in some circumstances, the use of drugs to induce regular bowel movements. Establishing a consistent bowel habit and addressing lifestyle variables can dramatically reduce constipation-related symptoms.

Variability and Intensity of Symptoms

One defining aspect of IBS is the heterogeneity in symptom presentation and severity. Symptoms can wax and wane, with patients having periods of relative symptom alleviation followed by flare-ups of heightened intensity. Understanding this diversity is vital for designing tailored management options that respond to the dynamic character of IBS.

The reasons for symptom aggravation can be various and include things such as stress, food choices, hormone cycles, and concomitant diseases. Tracking symptoms over time and recognizing trends helps individuals to predict and manage symptom variations efficiently.

The level of IBS symptoms can range from moderate, where persons can maintain their regular activities with minor disturbance, to severe, when symptoms considerably impact the quality of life. The unpredictability of symptom severity adds a degree of complication to managing IBS.

Healthcare practitioners play a vital role in engaging with persons with IBS to negotiate the complexity of symptom fluctuation and severity. Tailoring treatment programs to meet particular symptoms, giving information on self-management measures, and promoting open communication contribute to a complete approach to IBS therapy.

In the following sections, we will look into the demographic variables impacting IBS, the possible long-term effects of uncontrolled IBS, and recommendations for successful care and lifestyle adjustments. Understanding the entire impact of IBS extends beyond symptom treatment and involves the larger elements of physical and emotional well-being.

Facts About Irritable Bowel Syndrome (IBS)

Irritable Bowel Syndrome (IBS) is a prevalent gastrointestinal condition that affects millions of persons worldwide. This section seeks to give a complete overview of crucial information linked to the prevalence of IBS on a worldwide scale and the demographic aspects, such as age and gender, that play a vital role in forming the landscape of this illness.

Prevalence Worldwide

IBS is a prevalent digestive condition, that affects individuals across varied geographical locations and cultural backgrounds. The prevalence of IBS varies widely, with estimates showing that from 5% to 10% of the world's population develops symptoms associated with IBS. This makes IBS one of the most widespread gastrointestinal illnesses, underlining the need for heightened awareness, research, and appropriate management techniques.

Understanding the global incidence of IBS is vital for healthcare professionals, policymakers, and anyone looking to appreciate the magnitude of this ailment. While prevalence rates may fluctuate between nations, the overall burden of IBS on healthcare systems and quality of life is a shared problem.

Age and Gender Demographics

The effect of IBS extends beyond its incidence, delving into particular demographic characteristics that determine its occurrence. Examining age and gender demographics gives useful insights into the intricacies of IBS and informs focused approaches to care and education.

1. Age Groups Affected Most

IBS can present at any age, from childhood to late maturity. However, particular age groups are more typically impacted, and identifying these trends assists in early identification and management. Studies reveal that adults between the ages of 30 and 50 are more likely to get IBS. This key stage of adulthood is marked by different lifestyle variables, stresses, and physiological changes that may lead to the emergence or worsening of IBS symptoms.

The influence of IBS on different age groups goes beyond the physiological elements, incorporating social, professional, and family components. Younger persons may have difficulty in school settings and social relationships, while elderly folks may battle with the consequences of IBS on their daily routines and general well-being.

2. Gender Disparities

Gender discrepancies play a considerable influence in the frequency and expression of IBS. Research consistently suggests that IBS is more widespread in women than in males, with nearly twice as many women obtaining a diagnosis of IBS. This gender disparity raises fascinating issues concerning the interaction of hormonal, genetic, and psychological variables in the development and manifestation of IBS.

The causes for gender disparities in IBS remain a focus of continuing inquiry. Hormonal variations, particularly those connected with the menstrual cycle, are considered potential reasons for the greater occurrence of IBS in women. Additionally, societal variables and healthcare-seeking habits may impact the reporting and diagnosis of IBS across genders.

Understanding age and gender demographics in the context of IBS is crucial for customizing healthcare strategies and therapies. It allows healthcare practitioners to take a tailored strategy that recognizes the particular difficulties and demands of different demographic groups, creating a more effective and empathic delivery of treatment.

As we dive deeper into the multidimensional nature of IBS, the next parts will discuss the possible lifetime ramifications of uncontrolled IBS, techniques for successful management, and the critical role of a healthy lifestyle in minimizing the risk and effects of this ubiquitous gastrointestinal condition. By unraveling the layers of IBS, we seek to equip patients, caregivers, and healthcare professionals with the knowledge needed to negotiate the intricacies of this illness.

Lifetime Implications Without Proper Care

Irritable Bowel Syndrome (IBS), if left untreated, can have deep and lasting repercussions on an individual's life. In this part, we will look into the different ways in which the absence of effective treatment for IBS can damage the quality of life, contribute to psychological and emotional suffering, and potentially lead to difficulties that reach beyond the digestive system.

Impact on Quality of Life

One of the most immediate and pervasive implications of untreated or poorly managed IBS is the severe impact on an individual's overall quality of life. IBS symptoms, ranging from stomach discomfort to irregular bowel habits, can impair daily routines, social engagements, and professional responsibilities. The unexpected nature of IBS symptoms adds an element of uncertainty and stress to several parts of life.

Individuals with untreated IBS may find themselves facing obstacles in keeping a regular job schedule, participating in social gatherings, and even engaging in ordinary everyday chores. The dread of abrupt symptoms, such as urgent toilet trips or stomach discomfort, may lead to a reluctance to move far from familiar situations, further reducing one's quality of life.

Beyond the physical discomfort, the ongoing treatment of IBS symptoms may add to weariness and exhaustion. Coping with the unexpected nature of the disease can be emotionally exhausting, reducing energy levels and general well-being. As a result, individuals may report a reduced sense of vigor and excitement for life.

Psychological and Emotional Effects

The tight relationship between the stomach and the brain, frequently referred to as the gut-brain axis, highlights the significant psychological and emotional impacts of IBS. Chronic, untreated IBS can lead to heightened levels of tension, anxiety, and even depression. The chronic nature of gastrointestinal problems might lead to a sense of frustration, powerlessness, and isolation.

Individuals with IBS may find themselves engaged in a cycle where the stress of controlling symptoms exacerbates the symptoms themselves, causing a feedback loop of physical and mental anguish. Anxiety about probable flare-ups and the impact of IBS on everyday life might further contribute to an impaired mental health status.

The psychological toll of IBS extends to interpersonal relationships as well. Family members, friends, and coworkers may struggle to grasp the unseen obstacles encountered by those with IBS. This lack of understanding can contribute to feelings of isolation and alienation, exacerbating the emotional weight borne by individuals afflicted.

Potential Complications

While IBS is typically considered a functional gastrointestinal condition without substantial anatomical abnormalities, chronic and severe instances may lead to possible consequences. These issues can spread beyond the digestive system and damage other aspects of health.

1. Malnutrition: Chronic symptoms of IBS, particularly diarrhea and malabsorption difficulties, may contribute to nutritional deficits. Over time, this can lead to malnutrition, impairing the body's capacity

to receive needed nutrients for proper functioning.

2. Increased Healthcare Utilization: Untreated IBS generally leads to numerous healthcare visits, diagnostic testing, and consultations. The cumulative impact of healthcare use not only exerts a strain on the person but also on healthcare systems.

3. Impact on Sleep Patterns: The interruption produced by IBS symptoms, especially at bedtime, might contribute to sleep abnormalities. Poor sleep quality, if prolonged, may lead to several health conditions, including exhaustion, poor cognitive performance, and weakened immunological function.

4. worsening of Existing diseases: Individuals with pre-existing diseases, such as inflammatory bowel disease (IBD) or chronic fatigue syndrome, may experience worsening of their symptoms when IBS is left unmanaged. The interaction between different health issues underlines the significance of comprehensive care.

Recognizing the long-term ramifications of untreated IBS highlights the vital need for proactive and comprehensive care solutions. In the following sections, we will discuss successful techniques for controlling and minimizing the burden of IBS, integrating both medicinal therapies and lifestyle adjustments. By addressing the many components of IBS care, patients may recover control over their lives and work towards maximizing their overall well-being.

Management of Irritable Bowel Syndrome (IBS)

Irritable Bowel Syndrome (IBS) care entails a thorough and tailored approach, including the varying nature of symptoms and their impact on everyday life. In this part, we will discuss the essential features of IBS management, from finding a good diagnosis to adopting a range of treatment measures, including medicines, dietary modifications, and stress management approaches.

Diagnosis and Seeking Medical Help

The first step in effective IBS therapy is receiving a comprehensive diagnosis. While IBS is a functional condition without detectable anatomical abnormalities, a healthcare provider can make a diagnosis based on the presence and pattern of symptoms. It is vital for anyone having gastrointestinal difficulties to get medical care soon.

Healthcare practitioners may do a full medical history review, perform physical examinations, and prescribe specialized testing to rule out other potential causes of symptoms. These tests may include blood tests, stool testing, and imaging examinations. The procedure of diagnosis not only verifies the presence of IBS but also helps exclude other gastrointestinal diseases that may require alternative treatment options.

Seeking medical care early in the course of symptoms enables prompt intervention and the formulation of an effective management plan customized to the individual's needs.

Importance of an Individualized Treatment Plan

IBS presents differently in each individual, with symptoms ranging in form and degree. Therefore, the formulation of a tailored treatment plan is crucial for optimal management. A healthcare specialist, frequently a gastroenterologist, works closely with the patient to identify their individual symptoms, triggers, and lifestyle variables.

The tailored treatment strategy may involve a mix of medicines, dietary adjustments, and lifestyle changes. This individualized approach respects the unique elements of each person's experience with IBS and strives to address their specific issues.

Medications for Symptom Relief

Several drugs can give symptom alleviation for patients with IBS. The choice of medicine relies on the major symptoms reported by the individual.

1. Antispasmodic drugs: These drugs act to reduce stomach cramps and discomfort by relaxing the muscles of the gut. They might be particularly effective for persons with IBS-D (diarrhea-predominant IBS).

2. Anti-diarrheal drugs: For patients with IBS-D, anti-diarrheal drugs may be given to assist control of bowel movements and minimize diarrhea bouts.

3. Laxatives for Constipation: Individuals with IBS-C (constipation-predominant IBS) may benefit from the use of laxatives to produce regular bowel movements.

The choice of medicine is selected by the healthcare professional based on the unique symptom profile and individual response to therapy.

Dietary Changes

Diet plays a crucial part in controlling IBS symptoms. Several dietary regimens have demonstrated success in lowering symptoms and increasing overall gut health.

1. Low-FODMAP Diet: FODMAPs (fermentable oligosaccharides, disaccharides, monosaccharides, and polyols) are particular kinds of carbohydrates that might cause IBS symptoms. The low-FODMAP diet involves decreasing the intake of certain carbs to reduce symptoms.

2. Fiber consumption: Adequate fiber consumption is vital for maintaining bowel regularity. For those with IBS, soluble fiber sources, such as oats and psyllium, may be particularly useful.

3. Probiotics: Probiotics are living bacteria that give health advantages when taken in suitable doses. They can contribute to intestinal health and may help ease certain IBS symptoms. Probiotics can be received through food sources or supplementation.

Stress Management Techniques

The gut-brain axis, which symbolizes the bidirectional link between the stomach and the brain, highlights the role of stress on IBS symptoms. Stress management approaches can play a crucial role in minimizing the frequency and intensity of symptoms.

1. Mindfulness & Meditation: Practices such as mindfulness meditation create a heightened awareness of the present

moment, increasing relaxation and lowering stress levels. Mindfulness-based stress reduction (MBSR) programs have demonstrated efficacy in controlling IBS symptoms.

2. Relaxation Exercises: Techniques such as deep breathing, gradual muscle relaxation, and guided visualization can assist individuals manage stress and limit its influence on gastrointestinal function.

Incorporating stress management into the entire treatment strategy emphasizes the interconnection of physical and mental well-being in the context of IBS.

The effective therapy of Irritable Bowel Syndrome includes a holistic approach that incorporates the unique elements of each individual's experience. Seeking an early diagnosis, devising a tailored treatment plan, and including medicines, dietary modifications, and stress management strategies are key components of a holistic strategy. By addressing the different variables contributing to IBS symptoms, individuals can acquire better control over their illness and work towards improving their overall quality of life.

Healthy Lifestyle and Behaviors to Reduce Risk

Adopting a healthy lifestyle is increasingly acknowledged as a significant element in minimizing the risk of numerous health disorders, and Irritable Bowel Syndrome (IBS) is no exception. In this part, we look into study findings that show the relationship between lifestyle choices and IBS risk, stressing prominent beneficial habits that can play a crucial role in lowering the possibility of acquiring this gastrointestinal condition.

Research Findings on Lifestyle and IBS

Recent research has shed light on the association between lifestyle variables and the occurrence of IBS. Understanding these facts can empower individuals to make educated decisions that enhance digestive health and perhaps lower the likelihood of getting IBS.

Research, such as the research performed by Vincent Chi-ho Chung from the Chinese University of Hong Kong, reveals a substantial link between a healthy lifestyle and a decreased risk of IBS. The study, which evaluated over 64,000 individuals in the United Kingdom, discovered crucial habits that were highly connected to keeping a IBS at bay. These habits included not smoking, engaging in rigorous exercise, obtaining adequate sleep, keeping a high-quality balanced diet, and exercising moderate alcohol use.

By adopting one or more of these practices, people displayed a decreased chance of acquiring IBS. The research stressed the possibility of lifestyle adjustment not only in controlling IBS symptoms but also in avoiding the emergence of the disorder.

Notable Healthy Behaviors

1. Not Smoking:
Not smoking appeared as a key factor in lowering the incidence of IBS. The study by Chung et al. revealed a 14% decreased

incidences of IBS in persons who never smoked. This discovery adds to the various health advantages linked with a smoke-free lifestyle.

The particular pathways connecting smoking and IBS risk are not fully explored, however, it is well-established that smoking can have deleterious impacts on gastrointestinal health. From an IBS viewpoint, avoiding smoking appears as a real and powerful method to increase digestive well-being.

2. Regular Exercise:
Vigorous exercise, another cornerstone of a healthy lifestyle, exhibited a robust connection with a decreased incidence of IBS. The study indicated a 17% decreased

risk in persons with high levels of intense physical exercise.

Exercise has diverse advantages for general health, and its good influence on the digestive system is well-documented. Physical exercise improves regular bowel movements, decreases stress, and boosts the overall function of the gastrointestinal system. Incorporating regular exercise into one's routine appears as a proactive technique to decrease IBS risk.

3. Adequate Sleep:
Quality sleep is increasingly regarded as a cornerstone of good health, and its significance in digestive well-being is no exception. The study showed a 27%

decreased incidence of IBS in persons receiving at least 7 hours of sleep each night.

Sleep deprivation can affect the precise balance of hormones that drive hunger, stress response, and gut function. Ensuring enough and restful sleep benefits not just IBS risk reduction but also general physical and mental well-being.

4. Healthy Diet Choices:
The relevance of a high-quality balanced diet in lowering IBS risk cannot be emphasized. The findings underlined the beneficial relationship between a healthy diet and decreased IBS incidence. Specific dietary treatments, such as the low-FODMAP diet, have attracted attention

for their potential in controlling IBS symptoms.

Embracing a diet rich in fiber, whole grains, fruits, and vegetables while reducing the intake of identified triggers can contribute to digestive health. Working with healthcare specialists, particularly dietitians, can help individuals customize their dietary choices to their personal requirements.

5. Moderate Alcohol Consumption:
The study also emphasized moderate alcohol use as a factor linked with a decreased incidence of IBS. While the particular processes are not completely known, moderation in alcohol use accords with wider guidelines for overall health.

Excessive alcohol drinking can irritate the gastrointestinal tract and lead to digestive disorders. Adopting a thoughtful and cautious approach to alcohol use helps not just digestive health but also general well-being.

Incorporating significant healthy habits into one's daily appears as a proactive and evidence-based method to minimizing the risk of Irritable Bowel Syndrome. Not smoking, engaging in regular exercise, obtaining appropriate sleep, adopting good food choices, and practicing moderate alcohol use together contribute to a comprehensive strategy for supporting digestive well-being. As individuals become aware of these links and adopt these practices into their lives, they empower themselves to take responsibility for their health and perhaps minimize the chance of getting IBS.

Caregiving and Support for Individuals with IBS

Caring for patients with Irritable Bowel Syndrome (IBS) demands a complex and caring approach. In this part, we cover the essential role of caregivers, the value of providing a supportive atmosphere, effective communication tactics, and how to encourage good lifestyle choices for people facing the problems of IBS.

Understanding the Role of Caregivers

Caregivers play a key role in the well-being of patients with chronic diseases, and IBS is no different. Understanding the issues experienced by persons with IBS and the impact on their everyday lives is vital for caregivers to provide appropriate assistance.

Individuals with IBS may suffer a range of symptoms, from stomach discomfort and bloating to irregular bowel movements. These symptoms can range in strength and frequency, resulting in unexpected and often devastating bouts. Caregivers need to be alert to these variances and identify the particular requirements of each individual.

Additionally, IBS can have psychological and emotional ramifications, including stress, anxiety, and a possible impact on overall quality of life. Caregivers must approach their position with sensitivity, knowing the entire nature of well-being and realizing that emotional support is vital to controlling IBS.

Creating a Supportive Environment

Establishing a supportive atmosphere is vital for those with IBS. Caregivers may contribute greatly to establishing a place that encourages comfort, understanding, and a sense of security.

1. Understanding Triggers and Preferences: Caregivers should engage cooperatively with people to identify specific triggers that increase IBS symptoms and learn their preferences for managing pain. This may include nutritional considerations, stress management approaches, and lifestyle improvements.

2. Accommodating Dietary Needs:

Dietary choices have a key role in treating IBS symptoms. Caregivers can aid by providing access to items that correspond with dietary choices and constraints. This may entail meal planning, grocery buying, and creating a supportive culinary environment.

3. Flexible Schedules:

IBS symptoms can be unexpected, and individuals may demand flexibility in their daily routines. Caregivers may participate by keeping open communication and modifying routines when required to meet unanticipated obstacles.

4. Creating a Relaxing Space:

Stress can increase IBS symptoms, stressing the necessity of maintaining a quiet and relaxing atmosphere. Caregivers can contribute to this by introducing stress-reducing aspects into the living space, such as comfortable seating places, calming colors, and minimum clutter.

Communicating Effectively

Effective communication is a cornerstone of caregiving, especially when assisting persons with a chronic disease like IBS. Open and sympathetic communication creates understanding and supports a collaborative approach to tackling the problems offered by IBS.

1. Active Listening:

Caregivers should exercise active listening to appreciate the specific experiences and concerns of persons with IBS. This entails providing undivided attention, asking clarifying questions, and expressing empathy.

2. Encouraging Dialogue about Symptoms:

IBS symptoms may be sensitive subjects, and individuals may be hesitant to discuss them freely. Caregivers may provide a safe environment for communication by exhibiting openness, non-judgment, and a readiness to listen without imposing answers.

3. Collaborative Decision-Making:
In topics about lifestyle choices, treatment programs, and daily routines, caregivers and individuals should engage in joint decision-making. This method encourages individuals to actively engage in their treatment and provides a sense of autonomy.

4. Educating and Being Informed:
Caregivers should devote time to studying the basics of IBS, including its symptoms, causes, and potential management techniques. This understanding helps caregivers to provide educated assistance and contribute meaningfully to the decision-making process.

Encouraging Healthy Lifestyle Choices

Caregivers have a significant role in influencing and promoting good lifestyle choices for patients with IBS. Proactive actions can be done to integrate behaviors that contribute to general well-being and perhaps relieve symptoms.

1. Collaborative Meal Planning:
Dietary choices are crucial to treating IBS symptoms. Caregivers might engage in collaborative meal planning, considering individual preferences and constraints. This collaborative approach ensures that food choices are both helpful and pleasurable.

2. Promoting Physical Activity:

Regular exercise has been connected with a decreased incidence of IBS, and caregivers can encourage physical activity as part of a healthy lifestyle. This may entail engaging in activities together, such as walks or light workouts, based on individual capacities.

3. Stress Reduction Techniques:

Stress management is critical for patients with IBS, and caregivers may offer and support stress reduction practices. This may involve activities such as mindfulness, meditation, or relaxation techniques. Creating a peaceful and supportive atmosphere leads to stress reduction.

4. Facilitating Healthcare Engagement:
Caregivers can help persons find proper medical treatment and attend healthcare appointments. This engagement guarantees that healthcare personnel are constantly informed about the individual's condition and may change treatment strategies accordingly.

Caregiving for patients with IBS demands a comprehensive and empathic approach. Through comprehension of the distinct obstacles presented by IBS, the establishment of a nurturing atmosphere, proficient communication, and the promotion of health-conscious lifestyle decisions, caregivers can significantly contribute to the general welfare of individuals managing the intricacies of this gastrointestinal ailment.

Conclusion

In the path of understanding and managing Irritable Bowel Syndrome (IBS), we have dug into the subtleties of this gastrointestinal ailment, investigated its numerous features, and addressed techniques for complete care. As we close, it's necessary to repeat key topics and underline the need to take a holistic approach to treatment for patients with IBS.

1. Understanding IBS:

Irritable Bowel Syndrome is a complicated gastrointestinal illness characterized by symptoms such as stomach discomfort, bloating, diarrhea, and constipation. Its causes are numerous, encompassing elements like oversensitive nerves, stress, genetic susceptibility, and environmental effects.

2. Symptoms and Variability:

IBS symptoms vary greatly among individuals, both in terms of nature and degree. Abdominal discomfort, bloating, diarrhea, and constipation are frequent signs, and the diversity of symptoms underlines the complexities of controlling this illness.

3. Facts and Demographics:

IBS has a widespread prevalence, affecting up to 1 in 10 persons globally. It demonstrates age and gender differences, with particular age groups and females being more vulnerable. Understanding these demographics is vital for targeted treatment and assistance.

4. Lifetime Implications:

Without adequate management, IBS may drastically damage the quality of life. Beyond the physical symptoms, patients may endure psychological and emotional repercussions, and serious problems might occur if the illness is not well handled.

5. Management Strategies:

Diagnosis and obtaining medical care are key stages in controlling IBS. Individualized treatment strategies, including medicines for symptom alleviation, dietary adjustments, and stress management techniques, are critical components of effective therapy.

6. Healthy Lifestyle for Risk Reduction:
Research findings stress the relevance of a healthy lifestyle in minimizing the chance of getting IBS. Not smoking, regular exercise, proper sleep, good eating choices, and moderate alcohol intake together contribute to general well-being.

7. Caregiving and Support:
Caregivers play a significant role in assisting those with IBS. Creating a supportive atmosphere, good communication, and encouraging healthy lifestyle choices are critical parts of caring.

Emphasizing the Importance of Holistic Care

As we focus on the numerous elements of IBS, it becomes obvious that a holistic approach is important for optimal management and care. Holistic care embraces the interconnection of physical, emotional, and psychological well-being, realizing that one element impacts the other.

1. Individualized Treatment:
IBS appears distinctively in each individual, demanding tailored treatment strategies. Healthcare practitioners should consider not just the physical symptoms but also the emotional and psychological consequences of the disease when creating care solutions.

2. Addressing Emotional Well-being:

The emotional toll of IBS should not be underestimated. Stress, worry, and the impact on mental health are key components of the IBS experience. Holistic treatment entails embracing efforts to address emotional well-being, such as counseling, support groups, and stress reduction approaches.

3. Promoting Lifestyle Harmony:

Holistic treatment fosters a seamless integration of healthy lifestyle choices into everyday activities. This extends beyond controlling symptoms to building a lifestyle that fosters overall well-being. Caregivers and healthcare practitioners should work to encourage physical exercise, proper diet, and stress management.

4. Patient Empowerment:

Empowering individuals to actively engage in their treatment is a core concept of holistic management. This entails teaching patients about IBS, promoting open communication, and including them in decision-making processes. When individuals feel empowered, they are more likely to stick to treatment regimens and embrace healthy lifestyle behaviors.

5. Continuous Learning and Adaptation:

IBS is a dynamic condition, and successful therapy involves ongoing learning and change. Healthcare providers, caregivers, and individuals should be educated about developing research, treatment choices, and lifestyle changes. A proactive approach to learning to ensure that treatment stays current and relevant.

Caring for patients with IBS extends beyond managing immediate symptoms; it entails taking a holistic view that acknowledges the varied nature of the ailment. By recapitulating essential ideas and highlighting the need for holistic treatment, we want to educate patients, caregivers, and healthcare professionals toward an approach that increases the entire well-being of those navigating the challenges of Irritable Bowel Syndrome.

www.ingramcontent.com/pod-product-compliance
Lightning Source LLC
Chambersburg PA
CBHW050845260726
48660CB00006B/2449